L

DIGNITY
RESPECT
REDIRECT
PATIENCE

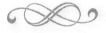

TOUCHED BY ALZHEIMER'S

AMY LESLEY

PAGE PUBLISHING, INC.
Conneaut Lake, PA

First originally published by Page Publishing 2020

ISBN 978-1-6624-0645-4 (pbk)
ISBN 978-1-6624-0646-1 (digital)

Printed in the United States of America

To my mother, my father, all of my beautiful children, my four-legged friend, Reggie, and the rest of my wonderful family

The material written in this book I experienced or learned through my twenty-two years of being a caregiver. Names have been changed for privacy and confidentiality.

Preface

Have you ever woken up in the morning from taking a nap and looked around for a minute but you didn't recognize your surroundings? Well, that's what a person with dementia or Alzheimer's sees. So if you start to notice signs like this with your loved one, you must remember: patience, reassurance, and lots of love.

Read up on Alzheimer's and your life and their lives might be made a lot easier, not perfect but better.

In my career, I have met so many beautiful and wonderful people and I also have lost so many. I have also had the joy and pleasure of knowing them.

It doesn't matter who you are. We are all special in our own way. We all hurt and feel pain in some way. People! We need to find a cure soon. It does not discriminate.

This is a prison none of us want to be in and the prison nobody walks out of.

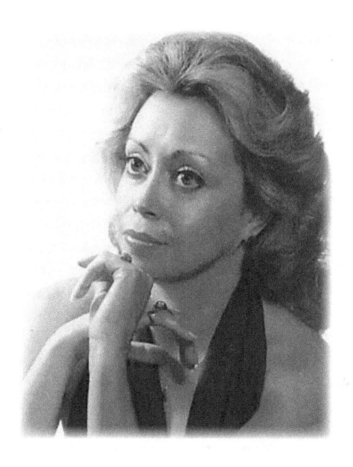

Life can be a challenge sometimes, but it's how we handle or accept each and every challenge for the outcome!

Some people that are facing this terrible disease with a loved one or friend choose to go on with their lives. Some choose to stay by the person's side. Both are all right. But just remember, never forget about your loved one or friend. Go whenever you can go to visit them. Give them a little love, time, and attention. This is for you both, you don't have to stay long. You will feel better for it, and so will they.

It is okay to go on with your life. Just always remember the ones left behind. Alzheimer's can happen to anyone. It doesn't care who you are. It puts you into a prison which goes from less offender to maximum offender in a matter of time. It is a thief that robs you of everything you love and cherish.

No one walks away from this prison.

1

Family

When we were growing up, my mother and father never taught us any differences in people. Everyone was treated the same. Mother said when she was young, her mother told her there were many different people in the world of many colors.

Red, yellow, brown, black, and white. In God's eyes, we are all the same, equal.

My parents, when they were a young couple, worked very hard to get where they were in life. They saved to buy their home, and when they did, they were overjoyed! Then they saved for an addition for the house—first the family room and extra bathroom, then the sunroom and patio, along with raising four children. It wasn't easy! It was their dream. When you come from humble beginnings, you try to do better for your family. Well, they did. When my father passed away, they had everything they needed. My father was always worried about whether they had enough money or not. So after he retired, he picked upside jobs gardening. Very seldom would he turn them down. Mom also worked very hard from being a glass girl at sixteen to being the manager. That is pretty good, I'll say. Along the way, they met a lot of nice people.

Mom is a very bright and smart woman. She will be ninety-five years old this year, and up until now, she would do her own banking and balancing of her checkbook. Now it's becoming a little confusing. She remembers the dresses she wore when she was a little girl and what color they were and what day and time she wore them. Then there are times she doesn't remember what she ate. There is a lot of repeating of what someone else has said. You might think that isn't bad, but if you knew my mother, she remembered everyone's names, actors, singers, and places she traveled.

Remember, these things or changes happen gradually. If you're not paying attention, you don't notice.

Back in the day, my great-aunt was a healer with natural herbs. People would go to her when they didn't feel well. We are blessed with many caregivers in our family.

I always say a lot of people are blessed with riches, but I think I'm the luckiest. I'm blessed with the love of my children and family. They are my gold.

My father's first episode was when he lost his way home in the neighborhood. He walked every day. He didn't recognize any of the streets or the direction he was going. Their little dog knew the way home, thank God. As it progressed, he became more and more paranoid. He used to know the people and the neighborhood like the back of his hand. Soon he stopped going for walks. He began looking out windows. He became suspicious of everyone. This wasn't like him. He did landscaping for a living. He was very much a people person. He was liked by everyone. Soon he started to hide behind the big trees in front of the house. Then he no longer wanted to go outside.

So at that point, we had to get home health to come in and help Mom with his ADLs, to assist him with getting ready for the day, brushing hair and teeth, washing up, and dressing. Dad wasn't going to allow it. As he progressed into this withdrawal from life, he began to fall more frequently. This was too much for Mom. So my sisters and I began alternating spending the night to help. We all had our own jobs to go to and children to take care of. Then the time came when Mom just couldn't do it anymore. So Daddy had to go to a nursing home. I went to see him.

Every day as I worked at the facility as a caregiver, Daddy would wait by the elevator, or he would look in the mirror facing the elevator and holler my name when he would see me. Dad was a very modest man; he didn't like being there, although he was treated very well. All of my coworkers just loved him! The care was above and beyond. Soon he stopped eating and talking and didn't want to leave the nursing home. Somebody from our family was always there with him. Mom was there every day. One day, he was sent to the hospital. He stayed a week and was sent back to the nursing home. That same month, he passed away! There has been a hole in my heart that will never close. If only I could have done more.

2

How It All Started

My choice to become a caregiver was made mainly because of all the wonderful people I've met in my life. There are so many that have nobody or no family to count on for daily tasks, like running them to doctor's appointments or just getting them groceries and, most of all, just someone to talk to. There was a time when I had my own business as a hairdresser. It was called "hair on the go." My choice was to go to the disabled and seniors. This was one of the best decisions I made in my life. I enjoyed my job bigtime! Just being able to see these wonderful people that welcomed you with open arms. For some, I would be the only person they would see or talk to for days. I would do what was called for that day—color, perms, haircuts, whatever they needed. They would tell me how they felt and about their story for the day. I think they enjoyed that more than anything. When I was finished, we would sit and have coffee and doughnuts. Then it would be time to leave. I would ask if they needed anything from the store.

I always felt bad taking their money, so I mostly broke even.

Then things started to fall apart. I became ill. I had to go to the hospital. So by the time I got out of the hospital, I had lost some customers. I was so sad.

That was one of the best jobs, and it was so rewarding.

So at the age of fifty, I decided to go back to school with my two daughters. They sort of "twisted my arm." I thought I was too old to learn, and guess what? I went on to get my CNA certification. *Wow*, I thought, *can I really do this?* Here I go on my new challenge. I studied very hard and passed with good grades. I started my new life as a certified nursing assistant. I applied for a job at a nursing home. I got the job. Boy, was I excited to start my new job! I started finding out that all of the people that worked there felt the same way about the seniors as I did. They were very caring, compassionate, and dedicated to the care and needs of the residents. When I say they all felt the same way, I mean all—from the laundry personnel to housekeeping, kitchen, and the DoN (director of nursing), as well as the director of the whole crew.

We all picked up for one another . The nurses would jump right in there and help their CNAs when needed, even the director of nursing. She wore a scrub top to work and was ready at all times. We had one another's backs. I loved working with each and every one of them. I learned so much from every one of you! Thank you!

A Day on the Job

Going to work was pure pleasure. People with dementia and Alzheimer's might not remember some things, but I'll tell you, when I worked in the unit, they knew my voice and did recognize me. Rise and shine, I would say as I walked down the hall. I started with the ones that were ready to get up and let the sleepyheads sleep longer, unless it was their shower day. This is the way my day started, unless we had a crisis. Then we would all work together and handle it.

Then it was on with the day. I would always bring in sweet rolls or cookies to have with coffee at snack time. After breakfast, we would wash up and take care of necessities. Then we would gather everyone to sit down and read the paper. Then if I had their attention, we would talk about their lives— what they did for a living, their families. Some would remember quite a bit and some only bits and pieces, but we were all involved.

Then it was snack time. Boy, that was the high-light of the day. After we sat and enjoyed coffee and sweets, it was time to take care of necessities, like bathroom and rest time.

The walkers, they are the residents that would walk constantly. They would walk up and down the long hallway into people's rooms. They just walk. So you see, it was quite a job just to get them to sit down or to give care, even to get them to participate in any activity. That's when reapproach came in.

After rest time, we would start getting the residents ready for lunch, assisting them again to the bathroom, and washing their face and hands, etc. Then we would sit them down for lunch. Some of the residents handled this very well themselves, while some needed our assistance. There were also some who refused. Again, this is where reapproach came in.

When they would refuse, we would turn to the next resident and try with them. You would work your way around the table until done. They usually wouldn't refuse all the time. It's just that they didn't have control of much anymore, so the things they can control, they do! Then you reapproach. You may have to do this more than once. But you can't give up because if you do, they won't get the nourishment they need. Don't get upset with them. Remember, patience!

After lunch was refresh time and then music, exercise, dancing, or a movie. Sometimes it was all of them. It depended pretty much on their energy level or how involved they were. Everyone has/had good and bad days.

4

The Unit

This is a lockdown unit. This is when you can't leave freely. Someone has to be with the resident at all times. The unit would hold up to sixteen residents at a time. A CNA would have to have special training to work in the unit because of the behaviors. All it would take was one to get everyone worked up. That's when they would get combative and attempt to hurt you or themselves. Walk slowly and approach the resident quietly and talk to that person in a clear, low voice and try to meet their needs. If they want to walk, walk with them. If they want to talk, talk with them. Remember, you are in their world. It's not about what you want; it's about what they want or need. In their world, things are very scary, and they are unsure of everything.

In the resident's world, everything has to stay the same. Furniture, for example, shouldn't be moved around. Their routine has to stay the same.

Remember, empathy, respect, dignity, and reassurance. Residents/patients love this! The right words go a long way.

If a situation starts to get too much to handle, put resident in a safe place and go to another room until they calm down and then attempt reapproach. It may take a lot of repetition with this disease process. At the end of the day, if you enter with an attitude, you will generally get attitude. If you enter with a calmness and understanding, you generally get calm. Remember, they are terrified inside. They are thinking, *Who is this person trying to tell me what to do? Who am I?* It becomes harder and harder for them to do their basic living tasks, like how to eat. They are being locked up in this body. How can this be? They are frequently on the defensive! Don't argue with them; it will only make the situation worse. This is their space, their home. Leave for a while but just make sure they will be safe. Get control and reapproach after a while. So again, patience, love, and respect will be what you bring into the room.

We can always attempt to make the resident's world a better place. Remember, they didn't choose to be in this life of not knowing who you are, where they are, who they are, or what's going on.

Most of the time, residents won't remember how or why they got where they are. Some have been dropped off by a family member, never to return. Please never do that! Explain to the person, even if you don't think they will understand. They deserve that much and more. Come back to see them. Maybe you can't visit every day, but that's okay; just come when you can. You might think they won't notice, but they will wait, just like everyone else. They may not remember why they are waiting, but when they see you, joy and a smile will come over their face. Also remember when a loved one goes deeper into their disease, please don't leave and never come back. They are hurting inside but have no understanding of why this is happening. One minute they are living life and in control, and then all of a sudden, things change and they have lost control a little at a time until there is none left. They may remember or come back for a minute or two. Wouldn't you want to be there if possible? Respect and love are key words. Life will always have its bumps and turns. We just don't know when they are coming!

You may notice your loved one sinking deeper. The sparkle is getting dimmer. You can't give up on them.

It can happen to anyone at any time!

5

Residents I've Had the Joy and Pleasure of Knowing

One of my residents, I will call her Molly, was very angry. She wouldn't eat or drink or talk to anyone. Obviously due to the fact that she wasn't eating, she was not getting any nutrients that she needed to survive. This was causing her skin to break down and have open sores. It was getting very bad and fast. So here I go—I always appreciate a good challenge! I would talk to her calmly every morning. "Good morning, Molly," I would say. "How are you today?"

No response. "It's a beautiful day out today." Her response was a grunt. Things continued this way for a day or two. Next, I tried to get her to drink a health shake, which wasn't going very well at first. So I told her if she would take one drink, I would leave her alone. So it started. And the next day, she took three sips, and so on. Soon I got her to eat a little, one bite at a time. Naturally, as she started to eat and drink again, it made her feel better.

I then was able to get her to sit up for a while. Day by day, she was getting a little better. The next morning, it was my day off. So she was looking for me, and my coworkers told her I was off. She asked if I was coming back, and they assured her that I was.

The very next day, I came into her room. I opened the drapes and said, "Good morning, Molly. It's going to be a good day today! We are going to sit up, eat a little something, and then we are going for a little ride."

She said, "Oh no!" She had not been down the hall or around the facility for some time. I said, "Oh, but it will be real nice to get out of bed and get some fresh air, stretch your legs, and meet some of your neighbors." She didn't want to meet anyone. Well, I won that round. So I washed her up, combed her hair, and helped dress her. This made her feel better, although she wouldn't admit it. Soon, she was up every morning, getting her nourishment, getting all cleaned up, and going for a ride, meeting and talking to the other residents.

Molly's skin had really improved. She did not have any family, so she was basically alone. We became her family. You see, that is our gift in return. If we can just improve the quality of life for that person in need. Molly had Alzheimer's. She didn't remember much. Again, this is where a lot of respect and love come into play.

Soon she would say, "Good morning, honey. How are you today?" I would reply, "Really good." She would then ask if we were going for a ride today! "We sure are," I would reply. She became one of the loveliest ladies I have had the pleasure of knowing. Once I gained her trust, she allowed me to assist her with her well-being and quality of life until she passed.

6

Mary

She was a beautiful tall blonde lady. She loved to dance and sing, and she just loved life. When her husband would come to visit, she would get so excited. She did remember his face and that he belonged to her, although she could not remember his name. They would sit and hold hands. When the music came on, she would get up and dance around.

He would sit and watch her and just smile. He would always come visit, heck or high water. They were so happy with each other.

Then as she progressed with Alzheimer's, she started to forget who he was. He would still come and visit just to be with her, hold her hand, and watch her dance around and sing. He would just watch her and smile with love in his eyes. It didn't matter to him that she didn't remember all of the good things they shared together, especially the love they shared. It was so heartwarming to witness the love these two people shared together. There is everlasting love in this world. I danced around with Mary on many days. She just smiled at me when she saw me coming. She has also passed.

7

Resident Bell

I remember a very jolly resident who loved to shop. The only thing was that she would go shopping in other resident's room. When things went missing, we would go to her room and look, and sure enough, there it would be. So we returned it to the rightful owner. She would get a little upset but she would get over it quick and go shopping again.

She would also pack her bag and wait for her son to come and pick her up to take her to California. Of course, he didn't know a thing about it. She was a cute little lady who liked getting her hair done and makeup on. After I was finished, she would ask, "How do I look?" My answer was always "You look beautiful, absolutely beautiful!" Her son did eventually come to take her to California.

8

My Ballerina

In her mind, she was a ballerina. She told all of us all about the competitions she was in. She was ninety-eight years old. Her story was, she had won a competition, and they had given the trophy to someone else. She was very frail but with a lot of spirit. She was always worried about her face and wrinkles (at ninety-eight). She would say, "Girls, never rub your eyes from inside out. Always pat them from the outside in to avoid wrinkles." She was missing some teeth, so she had to get dentures. So when she got them, she had a smile so beautiful. That was the happiest I had seen her. From then on, her makeup and hair had to be done every day. Then I came to find out she wasn't a ballerina at all. Her daughter said she hadn't danced a day in her life. She passed away at 102 years old. Now she can dance all she wants to in heaven!

9

Myra

She took a liking to my family when my father came to the nursing home. She would always hang around my daddy's room. Cute little lady, about four feet one. She couldn't speak a lot of English. She loved to put ribbons and pretty barrettes in her hair.

She would follow me from room to room and wait outside the door until I was done with the resident. To her, I really think she thought she was doing her job. She loved cookies and candy, so I would bring some to her, and she would say, "For me?" "Yes," I would say, "all for you."

When my father passed away, she packed all of her things and was ready to go. That was one of the most difficult times I had to deal with. My heart was breaking. After all, she thought she was family. So I had to tell her that she couldn't go. She had to stay! Now she was hurt. After a while, things got back to normal. She followed me around, and I brought her cookies and candy. We did our job. She was at the nursing home for a few years after my dad passed. She is also now in heaven.

10

Doug

We had a gentleman who was a businessman. Every morning when he got up, he would get dressed and have to have the newspaper and a cup of coffee—two sugars and cream, and I mean in that order. So that meant he had to have his own newspaper because he would tuck it under his arm for the rest of the day. He was up and dressed, ready for work every day like clockwork. His daughter would come and pick him up and take him to the park and sometimes lunch. It was an easy task for her but sometimes not. He always wanted to see his dogs and his home. This went on for some time until he was starting to get angry when things didn't go his way. It all came to a halt when he became combative, and they had trouble getting him to come back into the facility. The visits became less frequent until his wife passed away. His daughter still came to see him. At this point, he would holler at her and say things to make her cry because she couldn't take him out of there.

When I became sick with breast cancer, he was still in the nursing home. He had become a recluse and wouldn't come out of his room or eat anything. I sure hated not being there. Sometimes you feel that you are the only one that understands them. They become part of your family. You give them respect and love; you protect them and make sure they have what they need for the day. If we don't, who will? How could we not treat them like family?

Remember, because they don't remember you, it's time to start a new relationship with your loved one or your friend. Whether you're the one that gets them up in the morning or the one that brings the doughnuts, build that new relationship with them. But never not try. One day, they may look up at you and remember. They will smile and make eye contact. Savor that moment because it may be gone in a flash. Remember, they love you as much as you love them.

Also remember they are fighting a bigger battle. Alzheimer's is slowly taking everything they treasure and love. They may become a little combative at times, as they are frightened. The thief is taking everything they hold dear—memories of life, love, and their children.

You are going to be dealing with a new personality. Get to know this person. Don't try to make them remember what was. Instead, learn how to enjoy them now. If they remember life as it was, that is fine. Also, if they are still able to communicate with you, let them tell you their story and listen.

11

Alzheimer's Doesn't Discriminate

It will rob anyone of all of their memories of the life they knew—loved ones, names, faces. No one knows why this disease happens to different individuals, but this thief doesn't care who you are, where you are, or how rich or poor you are. It takes your life and tucks it somewhere in your brain forever! So if you are one of the unfortunate ones that Alzheimer's has touched, remember to treat this person with dignity, respect, a lot of patience, and a whole lot of love. This can happen to anyone; it doesn't discriminate.

Never leave your loved one alone if possible. Remember, they once loved you unconditionally. If it gets to be too much, then walk away for a bit. I know it's a hard job. I'm there, remember? Lots and lots of patience is required.

Play the music they love; they will remember. We can't choose our destiny. Never be ashamed of doing the right thing. Treat people the way you would want to be treated!

I'm just a caregiver for twenty-two years.
Nobody walks away from this prison.

Amy B. Valerio Lesley

Signs to look for:

1. Not wanting to be around other people
2. Trouble holding conversation
3. Words becoming unclear, notable to understand
4. Not remembering where they put things
5. Losing interest—combing hair, bathroom
6. Losing interest in eating and drinking
7. Not wanting to leave their area
8. Depression, confusion

These are only some of the things to look for, not all.

Without God by my side, I would not be here today! To God be the glory!

9 781662 406454